WEIGHT LOSS JUICE RECIPES BOOK

"Revitalize Your Journey: Nourishing Juice Recipes for Effective and Enjoyable Weight Loss"

Megan Addison

TABLE OF CONTENTS

INTRODUCTION

Welcome to a journey of transformation—a journey inspired by real struggles, real triumphs, and the simple power of making better choices. I'm not a fitness guru or a nutrition expert, just someone who found a path to weight loss that felt sustainable and satisfying. This book is about sharing that journey with you and introducing you to the world of weight loss through delicious and nourishing juices.

A few years ago, I found myself standing in front of the mirror, feeling the weight of frustration and a few extra pounds. I tried various diets and exercise routines, but nothing seemed to stick. Then, a friend shared a simple juice recipe that kickstarted a change in my life. It wasn't a magic potion, just a tasty and nutritious blend that made me realize healthy choices can also be enjoyable.

In this book, you won't find complicated formulas or hard-to-pronounce ingredients. Instead, I want to take you on a practical, down-to-earth exploration of weight loss through juicing. We'll navigate together through energizing breakfast blends, refreshing midday sips, satisfying snacks, nourishing lunches, rejuvenating dinners, and even a few guilt-free desserts.

But this isn't just a recipe book; it's a companion on your journey. I'll share tips, tricks, and a one-week detox plan to kickstart your efforts. So, whether you're a complete beginner or someone looking for fresh ideas, let's embark on this adventure together.

Now, I invite you to turn the page and discover the wonders that a simple, homemade juice can bring to your weight loss journey. It's time to make small changes that lead to big results. Cheers to a healthier, happier you!

Take the first step today. Your journey to a better you begins now.

Chapter 1: Getting Started - Essential Tools and Ingredients Tips for Successful Weight Loss Juicing

Welcome to the first steps of your weight loss juicing journey! Getting started is often the most crucial part, so let's break it down into simple, actionable steps.

Essential Tools:

1. Juicer: Invest in a good quality juicer. Whether it's a centrifugal or masticating juicer, choose one that suits your budget and preferences. Remember, it doesn't need to be the fanciest model; reliability and ease of use are key.
2. Cutting Board and Knife: Have a sturdy cutting board and a sharp knife for preparing your fruits and vegetables. A little prep work goes a long way in making the juicing process smoother.
3. Glass or Container: Get a collection of glass jars or containers to store your juices. They not only keep your creations fresh but also make it easy to grab a juice when you're on the go.

Essential Ingredients:

1. Fresh Produce: Choose a variety of fresh fruits and vegetables. Opt for colorful options to ensure a mix of vitamins and minerals. Leafy greens, citrus fruits, and vibrant berries are excellent choices.
2. Herbs and Spices: Experiment with herbs like mint, basil, and spices like ginger or turmeric to add flavor and extra health benefits to your juices.
3. Liquid Base: Water, coconut water, or unsweetened almond milk can be the base of your juices. These keep your concoctions hydrating without adding unnecessary sugars.

Practical Tips:

1. Start Simple: If you're new to juicing, begin with straightforward recipes. A basic green juice with spinach, cucumber, and apple is an excellent beginner's choice.
2. Prep in Batches: Spend some time washing, peeling, and chopping your ingredients in advance. Preparing batches can save time during the week and keep you on track.
3. Balance is Key: Aim for a balanced mix of fruits and vegetables to ensure you get a variety of nutrients. Too much fruit can add excess sugars, so find the right balance for your taste and health goals.

4. Experiment: Don't be afraid to try new combinations. Juicing is a creative process, and experimenting with different flavors can keep things interesting.

Getting started is all about simplicity and setting yourself up for success. Equip yourself with the right tools, choose fresh and colorful ingredients, and follow practical tips to make weight loss juicing a sustainable part of your routine. It's time to take that first step towards a healthier you!

Chapter 2: Understanding Nutrients - The Role of Nutrients in Weight Loss, Building Blocks of a Balanced Juice

Welcome to the heart of our weight loss juicing journey, where we'll unravel the essential role of nutrients and delve into crafting balanced, flavorful juices that nourish your body.

The Role of Nutrients in Weight Loss:

Vitamins and Minerals: These micro-powerhouses play a vital role in supporting your metabolism and overall well-being. Let's embrace the nutrient-rich world of fruits and vegetables to kickstart your weight loss.

Fiber: Nature's way of aiding digestion and keeping you satisfied, fiber is your ally in curbing those unwanted cravings. It's time to include fiber-packed ingredients to make your juices not only tasty but also filling.

Antioxidants: Think of antioxidants as your body's defenders against stress. Found abundantly in colorful fruits and veggies, they promote cellular health and support your body's natural defense mechanisms.

Building Blocks of a Balanced Juice:

Leafy Greens:

Practical Tip: Spinach is versatile and mild. Try a Spinach Citrus Boost:

2 cups fresh spinach

1 orange, peeled

1 cucumber, chopped

Water as needed

Colorful Fruits:

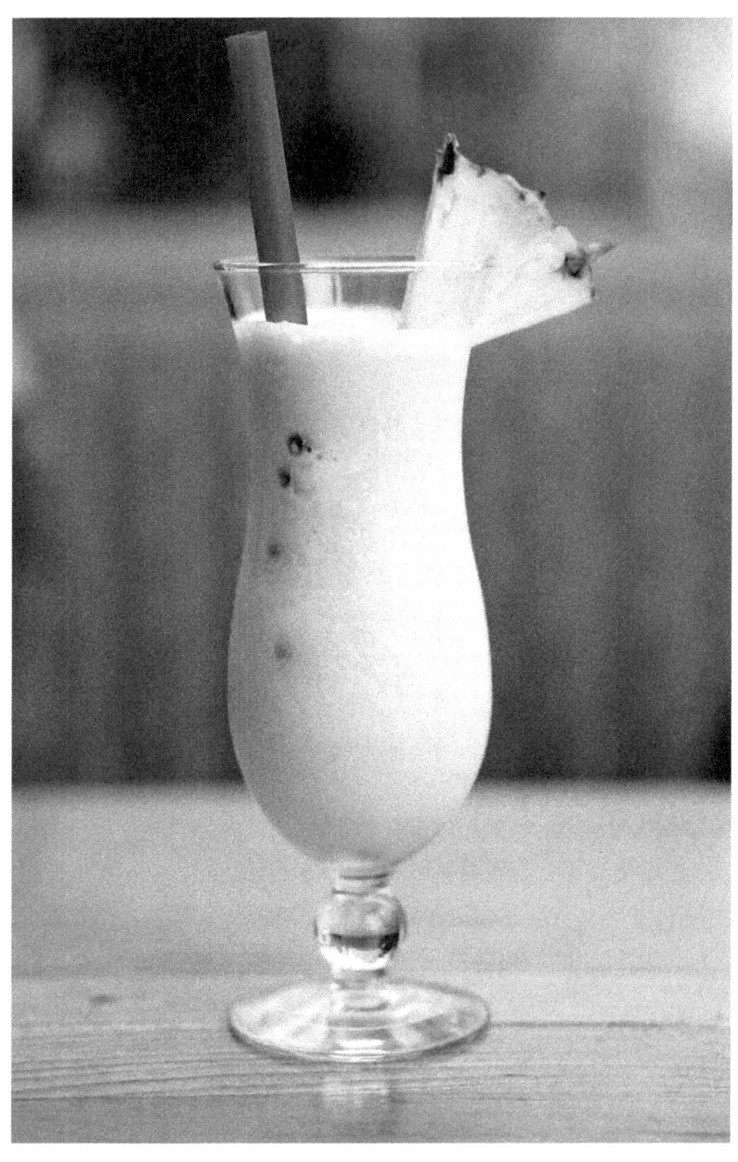

Practical Tip: Berries are not only rich in antioxidants but also delicious. Give the Berry Bliss a shot:

1 cup mixed berries (blueberries, strawberries, raspberries)

1 apple, cored

Handful of kale

Water as needed

Vegetables:

Practical Tip: Carrots bring sweetness and a dose of beta-carotene. Whip up a Carrot Ginger Zing:

4 carrots, chopped

1 apple, cored

Small piece of ginger

Water as needed

Liquid Base:

Practical Tip: Coconut water is hydrating and adds a subtle sweetness. Try a Tropical Green Delight:

Coconut water

Pineapple chunks

Handful of mint leaves

Water as needed

Many Recipes for Your Exploration:

Green Goddess Elixir:

2 cups kale

1 green apple, cored

1 cucumber, chopped

1 lemon, peeled

Water as needed

Citrus Splash Delight:

1 grapefruit, peeled

2 oranges, peeled

Handful of spinach

Water as needed

Beetroot Berry Boost:

1 small beetroot, peeled and chopped

1 cup mixed berries (blueberries, raspberries)

1 apple, cored

Water as needed

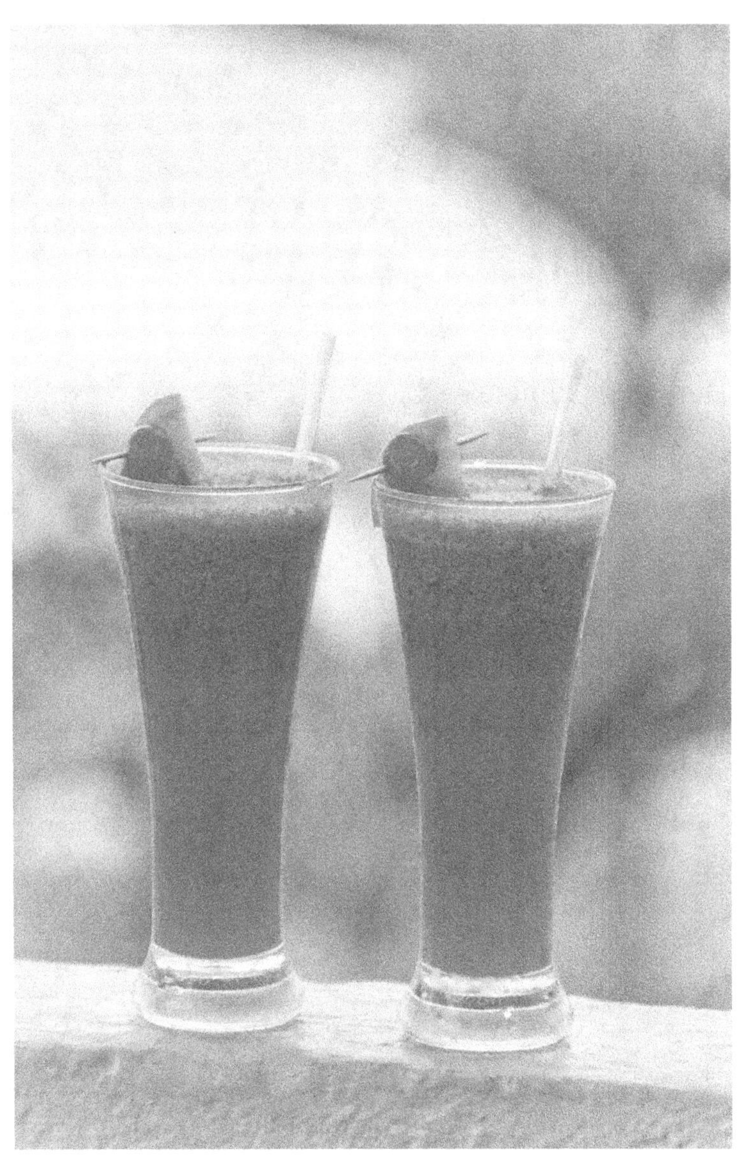

Minty Melon Refresher:

1 cup watermelon, cubed

1 cucumber, chopped

Handful of mint leaves

Water as needed

Experiment with these recipes, discovering the delightful world of nutrient-packed juices. The journey to a balanced, refreshing beverage that aids in your weight loss has just begun. Enjoy the flavors and the benefits as we continue this journey together!

Chapter 3: Energizing Breakfast Juices - Sunrise Citrus Boost, Berry Blast Morning Delight, Green Goodness Kickstart

Now, let's kickstart your day with the vibrant energy of breakfast juices. These recipes aren't just delicious; they're packed with the goodness you need to fuel your morning.

Sunrise Citrus Boost:

Practical Tip: Citrus fruits are rich in vitamin C, perfect for an immune boost.

1 orange, peeled

1 grapefruit, peeled

2 carrots, chopped

Water as needed

Berry Blast Morning Delight:

Practical Tip: Berries add a burst of antioxidants to your morning.

1 cup mixed berries (blueberries, strawberries, raspberries)

1 banana

Handful of spinach

Water as needed

Green Goodness Kickstart:

Practical Tip: Leafy greens provide essential nutrients without overpowering the flavor.

2 cups kale

1 green apple, cored

1 cucumber, chopped

1 lemon, peeledWater as needed

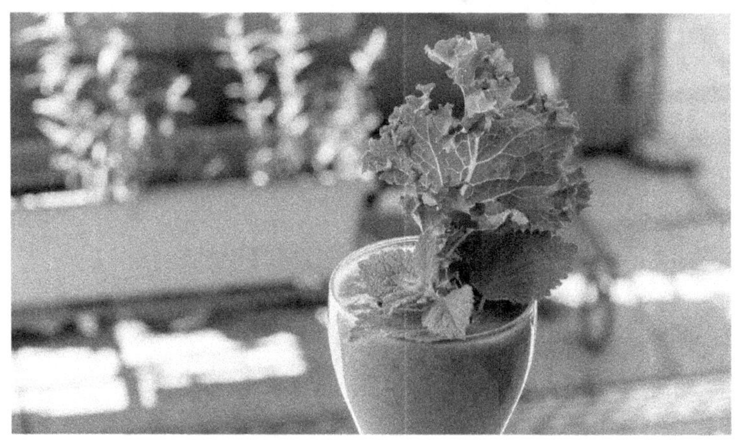

More Recipes for Your Breakfast Joy:

Tropical Morning Bliss:

Coconut water

1 cup pineapple chunks

1 kiwi, peeled

Handful of spinach

Water as needed

Apple Pie Delight:

2 apples, cored

1 teaspoon cinnamon

1 tablespoon chia seeds (optional)

Water as needed

Peachy Keen Sunrise:

2 peaches, pitted

1 orange, peeled

Handful of kale

Water as needed

Mango Banana Sunrise:

1 mango, peeled and pitted

1 banana

1 cup spinach

Water as needed

Practical Tips for Your Breakfast Juices:

Prep the Night Before: Chop fruits and veggies the night before to make your morning routine smoother.

Rotate Your Greens: Keep it interesting by rotating your leafy greens. Try spinach one day and kale the next.

Balance Sweet and Tangy: Experiment with the balance of sweet and tangy fruits to find the perfect flavor for your taste buds.

These breakfast juices aren't just about nutrition; they're about starting your day with a burst of freshness and vitality. Try these recipes and adapt them to suit your preferences. Here's to energized mornings and a healthier you!

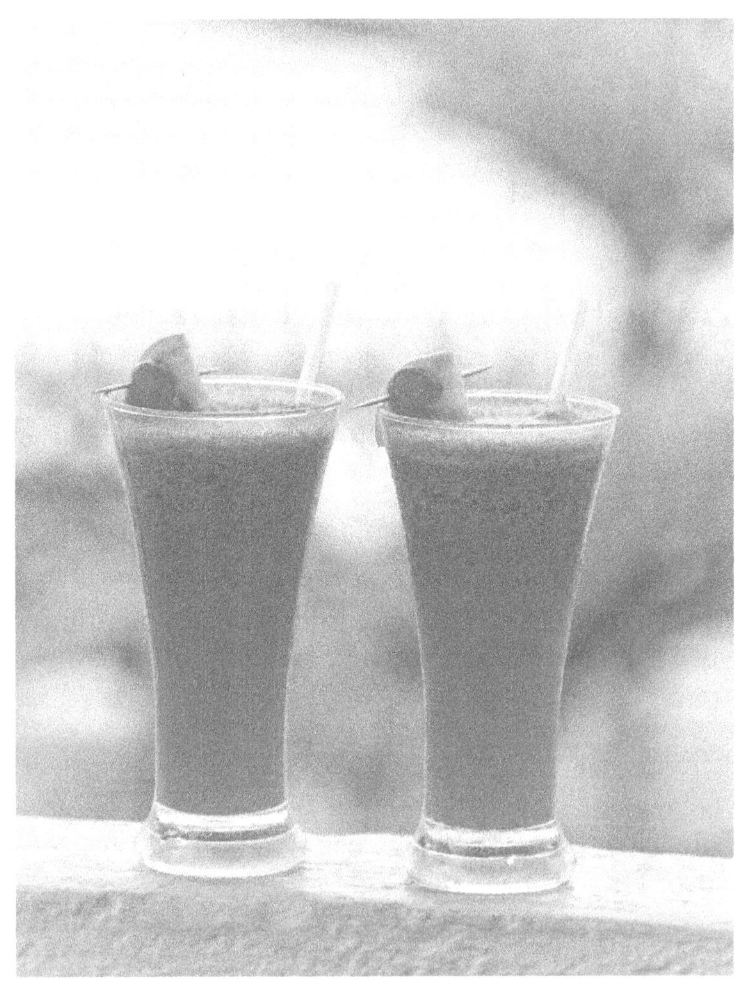

Chapter 4: Refreshing Midday Hydration - Cucumber Mint Cooler, Tropical Paradise Refresher, Watermelon Basil Bliss

As the day unfolds, let's keep the momentum going with refreshing midday hydration. These rejuvenating juices are not only hydrating but also a delightful break from your routine.

Cucumber Mint Cooler:

Practical Tip: Cucumbers are hydrating, and mint adds a burst of freshness.

1 cucumber, sliced

Handful of mint leaves

1 lime, peeled

Water as needed

Tropical Paradise Refresher:

Practical Tip: Pineapple and coconut water bring a taste of the tropics.

Coconut water

1 cup pineapple chunks

1 kiwi, peeledWater as needed

Watermelon Basil Bliss:

Practical Tip: Watermelon is not just sweet but also high in hydration.

2 cups watermelon, cubed

Handful of basil leaves

1 lemon, peeled

Water as needed

More Recipes for Your Midday Sip:

Citrus Mint Splash

2 oranges, peeled

Handful of fresh mint leaves

Water as needed

Ginger Lime Quencher:

1 inch ginger, peeled

2 limes, peeled

1 cucumber, sliced

Water as needed

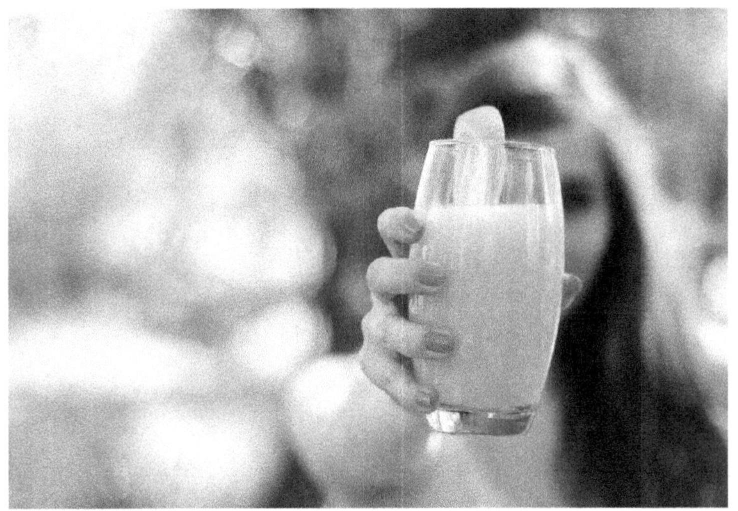

Pineapple Basil Breeze:

1 cup pineapple chunks

Handful of basil leaves

1 apple, cored

Water as needed

Mango Mint Bliss:

1 mango, peeled and pitted

Handful of mint leaves

1 lime, peeled

Water as needed

Practical Tips for Your Midday Hydration:

Experiment with Herbs: Herbs like mint, basil, and ginger can transform your midday hydration experience.

Adjust Water Content: Customize the water content to suit your preference. Some like it light, while others prefer a more concentrated flavor.

Use Chilled Ingredients: For an instant refresh, use chilled fruits and veggies or add ice cubes to your midday juices.

These midday hydration recipes are not just about drinking water; they're about enjoying a moment of refreshment and nourishment. Try these recipes, experiment with flavors, and find your favorite go-to midday pick-me-up. Here's to staying hydrated and feeling rejuvenated throughout the day!

Chapter 5: Satisfying Snack Juices - Apple Pie Delight, Carrot Cake Cravings, Creamy Green Avocado Dream

Let's transition to the world of satisfying snack juices—delicious blends that not only satiate your cravings but also provide a nutritious energy boost to keep you going.

Apple Pie Delight:

2 apples, cored

1 teaspoon cinnamon

1 tablespoon chia seeds (optional)

Water as needed

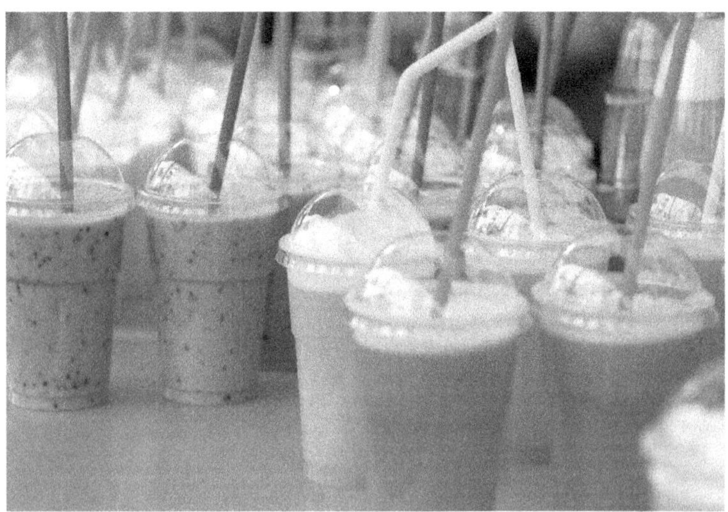

Carrot Cake Cravings:

Practical Tip: Carrots bring natural sweetness, and spices mimic the flavors of carrot cake.

4 carrots, chopped

1 apple, cored

1 teaspoon cinnamon

Water as needed

Creamy Green Avocado Dream:

Practical Tip: Avocado adds a creamy texture and healthy fats to keep you satisfied.

1 ripe avocado

Handful of spinach

1 green apple, cored

Water as needed

More Recipes for Your Satisfying Snack:

Banana Nut Bliss:

2 bananas

Handful of almonds

1 tablespoon flaxseeds (optional)

Water as needed

Berry Almond Crunch:

1 cup mixed berries (blueberries, strawberries, raspberries)

Handful of almonds

1 apple, cored

Water as needed

Peanut Butter Banana Delight:

2 bananas

2 tablespoons peanut butter

Handful of spinach

Water as needed

Orange Creamsicle Treat:

2 oranges, peeled

1/2 cup Greek yogurt

1 tablespoon honey (optional)

Water as needed

Practical Tips for Your Satisfying Snack Juices:

Add Protein: Include ingredients like nuts, seeds, or Greek yogurt to make your snack juices more satisfying.

Experiment with Spices: Spices like cinnamon, nutmeg, or vanilla can add depth to your snack juices.

Adjust Sweetness: Control the sweetness by adjusting the quantity of sweet fruits or adding a touch of honey if desired.

Satisfying snack juices are a tasty way to curb cravings and keep your energy levels steady throughout the day. Try these recipes, tweak them to your liking, and discover the joy of nutritious snacking. Here's to satisfying your cravings while staying on track with your wellness goals!

Chapter 6: Nourishing Lunch Blends - Lean Mean Green Machine, Beetroot Beauty Elixir, Quinoa Kale Power Punch

Let's elevate your lunchtime with nourishing blends that not only satisfy your taste buds but also provide the essential nutrients to power through the rest of your day.

Lean Mean Green Machine:

Practical Tip: This green powerhouse is excellent for a light and nutritious lunch.

2 cups kale

1 cucumber, chopped

1 green apple, cored

1 lemon, peeled

Water as needed

Beetroot Beauty Elixir: Practical Tip: Beetroot adds a vibrant color and is known for its potential health benefits.

1 small beetroot, peeled and chopped

1 apple, cored

1 carrot, chopped

Water as needed

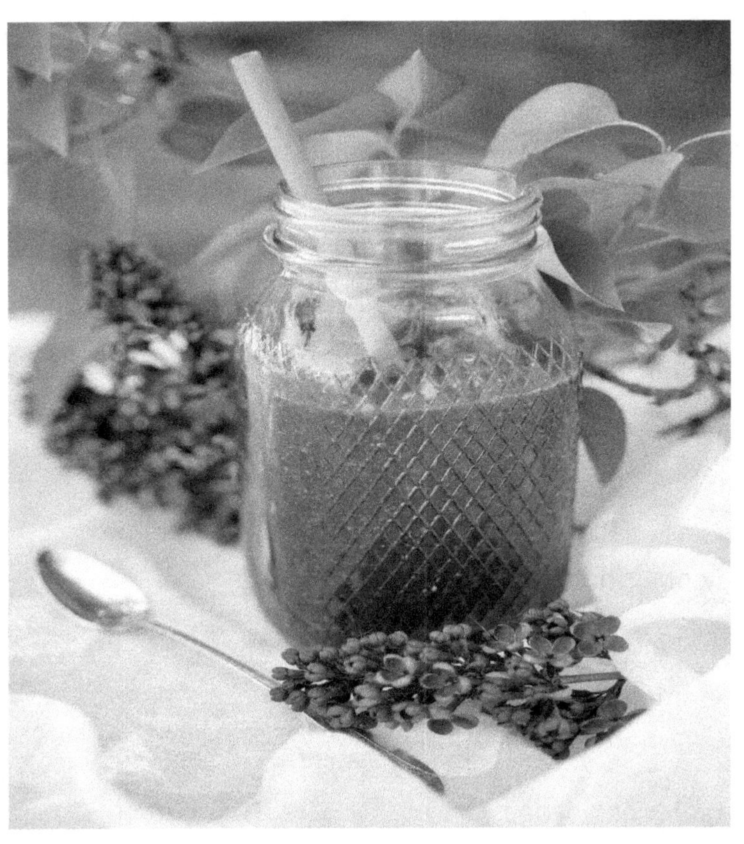

Quinoa Kale Power Punch:

Practical Tip: Adding cooked quinoa to your juice provides a source of protein and makes it more filling.

1 cup cooked quinoa

2 cups kale

1 cucumber, chopped

1 lemon, peeled

Water as needed

More Recipes for Your Nourishing Lunch:

Mango Avocado Bliss:

1 mango, peeled and pitted

1 ripe avocado

Handful of spinach

Water as needed

Tomato Basil Delight:

2 tomatoes

Handful of basil leaves

1 cucumber, chopped

Water as needed

Sweet Potato Spinach Powerhouse:

1 small sweet potato, cooked and peeled

2 cups spinach

1 apple, cored

Water as needed

Cabbage Crunch Booster:

2 cups cabbage, shredded

1 green apple, cored

1 lemon, peeled

Water as needed

Practical Tips for Your Nourishing Lunch Blends:

Include Protein: Incorporate ingredients like quinoa, avocado, or even Greek yogurt for added protein in your lunch juices.

Experiment with Vegetables: Don't shy away from veggies like cabbage, sweet potato, or tomatoes—they can add unique flavors and nutrients.

Prep Quinoa Ahead: Cook a batch of quinoa at the beginning of the week for quick and easy additions to your lunch blends.

Nourishing lunch blends are a delicious way to refuel and provide your body with the nutrients it needs. Try these recipes, customize them to your liking, and savor the goodness of a nourishing lunch that keeps you energized. Here's to lunchtime satisfaction and wellness

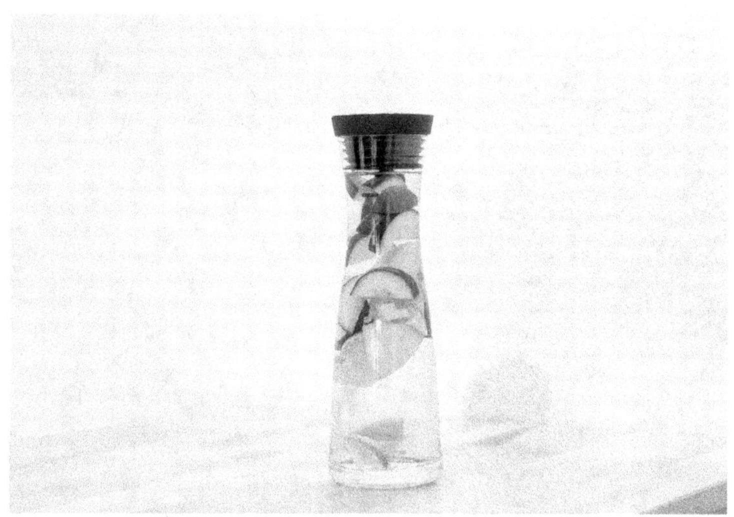

Chapter 7: Rejuvenating Dinner Juices - Spinach and Pineapple Cleanse, Tomato Basil Immunity Booster, Lemon Garlic Detoxifier

As the day winds down, let's focus on rejuvenating dinner juices that not only soothe your senses but also provide a dose of goodness to support your body's recovery during the night.

Spinach and Pineapple Cleanse:

Practical Tip: Spinach and pineapple combine for a refreshing and cleansing blend.

2 cups spinach

1 cup pineapple chunks

1 cucumber, choppe

Water as needed

Tomato Basil Immunity Booster:

Practical Tip*:* Tomatoes and basil team up for a flavorful juice loaded with immune-boosting properties.

3 tomatoes

Handful of basil leaves

1 carrot, chopped

Water as needed

Lemon Garlic Detoxifier:

Practical Tip*:* The dynamic duo of lemon and garlic aids in detoxification.

1 lemon, peeled

2 cloves garlic

1 cucumber, chopped

Water as needed

More Recipes for Your Rejuvenating Dinner:

Cucumber Mint Relaxer:

1 cucumber, sliced

Handful of mint leaves

1 lime, peeled

Water as needed

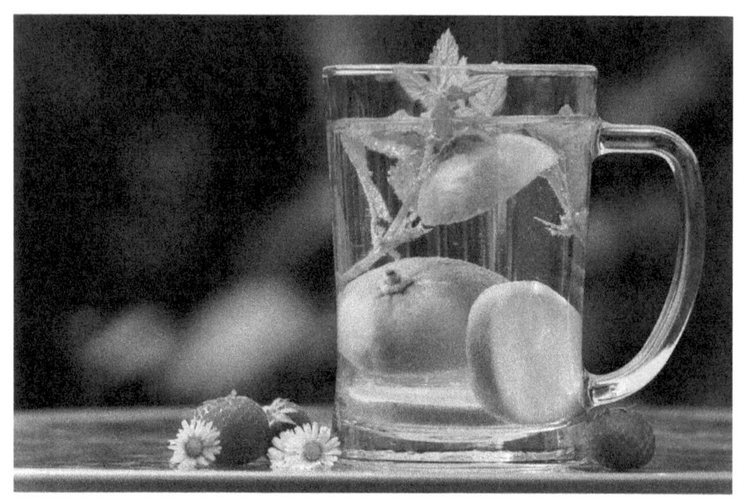

Avocado Tomato Twilight:

1 ripe avocado

2 tomatoes

Handful of spinach

Water as needed

Carrot Ginger Soother:

4 carrots, chopped

Small piece of ginger

1 apple, cored

Water as needed

Beetroot Citrus Serenity:

1 small beetroot, peeled and chopped

2 oranges, peeled

Handful of kale

Water as needed

Practical Tips for Your Rejuvenating Dinner Juices:

Opt for Lighter Ingredients: Keep your dinner juices light with ingredients like cucumber, spinach, and citrus fruits to aid digestion.

Include Detoxifying Elements: Ingredients like lemon, garlic, and ginger are known for their detoxifying properties—perfect for a rejuvenating dinner.

Stay Hydrated: Ensure your dinner juices have a good water content to support hydration, especially important as you prepare for a night of rest.

Rejuvenating dinner juices are a wonderful way to conclude your day on a healthy note. Try these recipes, adjust them to your taste, and embrace the nourishing power of dinner blends. Here's to a relaxing and revitalizing evening routine for a well-balanced lifestyle!

Chapter 8: Decadent Dessert Juices - Chocolate Banana Indulgence, Berry Cheesecake Delight, Mango Coconut Dream

Indulge your sweet tooth with dessert juices that not only satisfy your cravings but also infuse a burst of fruity decadence. Let's explore delightful blends perfect for those moments when you want a healthy yet indulgent treat.

Chocolate Banana Indulgence:

Practical Tip: Cacao nibs add a touch of chocolatey goodness without the excess sugar.

2 bananas

1 tablespoon cacao nibs

1 tablespoon almond butter

Water as needed

Berry Cheesecake Delight:

Practical Tip: Greek yogurt adds a creamy texture reminiscent of cheesecake.

1 cup mixed berries (blueberries, strawberries, raspberries)

1 banana

1/2 cup Greek yogurt

Water as needed

Mango Coconut Dream:

Practical Tip: Coconut water and mango create a tropical paradise in a glass.

Coconut water

1 ripe mango, peeled and pitted

Handful of shredded coconut

Water as needed

More Recipes for Your Decadent Dessert Juices:

Pineapple Mint Sorbet:

1 cup pineapple chunks

Handful of mint leaves

1 lime, peeled

Water as needed

Vanilla Almond Bliss:

1 teaspoon vanilla extract

Handful of almonds

1 banana

Water as needed

Peach Cobbler Fantasy:

2 peaches, pitted

1 teaspoon cinnamon

1 tablespoon chia seeds (optional)

Water as needed

Strawberry Shortcake Euphoria:

1 cup strawberries, hulled

1 banana

1 tablespoon honey (optional)

Water as needed

**Practical Tips for Your Decadent Dessert
Juices**:

Experiment with Sweeteners: Adjust sweetness with
natural alternatives like honey, agave, or maple
syrup.

Incorporate Nuts: Nuts add a delightful crunch and
healthy fats to your dessert juices.

Freeze Fruits: Use frozen fruits for a chilled, sorbet-
like consistency.

Decadent dessert juices are a guilt-free way to enjoy
the sweetness of life. Try these recipes, customize
them to your liking, and savor the joy of a healthy
dessert that delights your taste buds. Here's to guilt-
free indulgence and the simple pleasure of a sweet
ending!

Chapter 9: Tailored Plans for Weight Loss - One-Week Detox Plan, Monthly Transformation Challenge

Embark on a personalized journey toward your weight loss goals with practical plans designed to fit seamlessly into your lifestyle. Let's explore a one-week detox plan and a monthly transformation challenge, offering you a roadmap to a healthier, more vibrant you.

One-Week Detox Plan:

Practical Tip: Kickstart your detox journey with hydrating green juices and nutrient-packed blends.

Day 1: Green Beginnings

Spinach and Pineapple Cleanse

Cucumber Mint Relaxer

Day 2: Citrus Boost

Sunrise Citrus Boost

Lemon Garlic Detoxifier

Day 3: Berry Refresh

Berry Cheesecake Delight

Berry Almond Crunch

Day 4: Tropical Infusion

Tropical Paradise Refresher

Mango Coconut Dream

Day 5: Rooted Goodness

Carrot Cake Cravings

Beetroot Citrus Serenity

Day 6: Leafy Green Reset

Lean Mean Green Machine

Avocado Tomato Twilight

Day 7: Sweet Farewell

Chocolate Banana Indulgence

Peach Cobbler Fantasy

Monthly Transformation Challenge:

Practical Tip: Introduce variety with a mix of energizing breakfast juices, satisfying snack blends, nourishing lunch juices, rejuvenating dinner blends, and decadent dessert juices throughout the month.

Week 1: Breakfast Boost

Energizing Breakfast Juices

Week 2: Midday Recharge

Refreshing Midday Hydration

Week 3: Lunchtime Nourishment

Nourishing Lunch Blends

Week 4: Evening Renewal

Rejuvenating Dinner Juices

Bonus: Weekend Treat

Decadent Dessert Juices

Practical Tips for Your Tailored Weight Loss Plans:

Stay Hydrated: Drink plenty of water throughout the day to enhance the benefits of your weight loss journey.

Listen to Your Body: Pay attention to how your body responds to different ingredients and adjust your plans accordingly.

Meal Prepping: Prepare ingredients in advance to make the execution of your plans more convenient.

Tailored weight loss plans provide structure while allowing flexibility to suit your preferences. Experiment with these recipes, find what works best for you, and enjoy the transformative journey toward a healthier lifestyle. Here's to your well-deserved success in achieving your weight loss goals!

Chapter 10: Lifestyle Tips for Sustainable Results
- Incorporating Juicing into Daily Life, Staying
Motivated on Your Weight Loss Journey

As you embrace a healthier lifestyle, it's essential to
seamlessly integrate juicing into your daily routine
while maintaining motivation on your weight loss
journey. Let's explore practical tips for sustainable
results that fit into your lifestyle effortlessly.

Incorporating Juicing into Daily Life:

Practical Tip: Make juicing a convenient and
enjoyable part of your routine with these simple
strategies.

Morning Ritual:

Start your day with an energizing breakfast juice,
like the Sunrise Citrus Boost or Energizing Breakfast
Juices.

Prep ingredients the night before for a quick
morning blend.

Midday Pick-Me-Up:

Keep refreshing midday hydration options, such as Cucumber Mint Relaxer or Refreshing Midday Hydration, readily available.

Invest in a portable blender for on-the-go juicing convenience.

Workday Boost:

Incorporate nourishing lunch blends like Nourishing Lunch Blends or Lean Mean Green Machine into your workday.

Share your favorite recipes with colleagues to create a supportive juicing community.

Evening Relaxation:

Wind down with rejuvenating dinner juices such as Rejuvenating Dinner Juices or Lean Mean Green Machine.

Use calming herbs like mint or chamomile to enhance evening blends.

Staying Motivated on Your Weight Loss Journey:

Practical Tip: Maintain motivation with these practical and effective strategies.

Set Realistic Goals:

Define achievable short-term and long-term goals for your weight loss journey.

Celebrate small victories along the way to stay motivated.

Create a Support System:

Share your goals with friends or family members for encouragement.

Join online communities or forums to connect with others on similar journeys.

Variety is Key:

Experiment with a variety of recipes to keep your taste buds engaged.

Rotate different fruits and vegetables to ensure a diverse nutrient intake.

Track Your Progress:

Keep a journal to track your daily juicing habits and reflect on your journey.

Take regular measurements or photos to visually see your progress.

Practical Tips Recap:

Start Fresh Each Day: Begin your mornings with a rejuvenating juice.

Prepare Ahead: Prepping ingredients in advance makes juicing a breeze.

Stay Consistent: Create a routine that aligns with your lifestyle for long-term success.

Find Joy in the Journey: Celebrate the positive changes, no matter how small.

Incorporating juicing into your daily life and maintaining motivation are vital components of sustainable weight loss. Try these tips, customize them to fit your preferences, and enjoy the journey toward a healthier and more vibrant you. Here's to a sustainable and successful lifestyle transformation!

Chapter 10: Lifestyle Tips for Sustainable Results - Incorporating Juicing into Daily Life, Staying Motivated on Your Weight Loss Journey

As you embrace a healthier lifestyle, it's essential to seamlessly integrate juicing into your daily routine while maintaining motivation on your weight loss journey. Let's explore practical tips for sustainable results that fit into your lifestyle effortlessly.

Incorporating Juicing into Daily Life:

Practical Tip: Make juicing a convenient and enjoyable part of your routine with these simple strategies.

Morning Ritual:

Start your day with an energizing breakfast juice, like the Sunrise Citrus Boost or Energizing Breakfast Juices.

Prep ingredients the night before for a quick morning blend.

Midday Pick-Me-Up:

Keep refreshing midday hydration options, such as Cucumber Mint Relaxer or Refreshing Midday Hydration, readily available.

Invest in a portable blender for on-the-go juicing convenience.

Workday Boost:

Incorporate nourishing lunch blends like Nourishing Lunch Blends or Lean Mean Green Machine into your workday.

Share your favorite recipes with colleagues to create a supportive juicing community.

Evening Relaxation:

Wind down with rejuvenating dinner juices such as Rejuvenating Dinner Juices or Lean Mean Green Machine.

Use calming herbs like mint or chamomile to enhance evening blends.

Staying Motivated on Your Weight Loss Journey:

Practical Tip: Maintain motivation with these practical and effective strategies.

Set Realistic Goals:

Define achievable short-term and long-term goals
for your weight loss journey.

Celebrate small victories along the way to stay
motivated.

Create a Support System:

Share your goals with friends or family members for
encouragement.

Join online communities or forums to connect with
others on similar journeys.

Variety is Key:

Experiment with a variety of recipes to keep your
taste buds engaged.

Rotate different fruits and vegetables to ensure a
diverse nutrient intake.

Track Your Progress:

Keep a journal to track your daily juicing habits and reflect on your journey.

Take regular measurements or photos to visually see your progres

Practical Tips Recap:

Start Fresh Each Day: Begin your mornings with a rejuvenating juice.

Prepare Ahead: Prepping ingredients in advance makes juicing a breeze.

Stay Consistent: Create a routine that aligns with your lifestyle for long-term success.

Find Joy in the Journey: Celebrate the positive changes, no matter how small.

Incorporating juicing into your daily life and maintaining motivation are vital components of sustainable weight loss. Try these tips, customize them to fit your preferences, and enjoy the journey toward a healthier and more vibrant you. Here's to a sustainable and successful lifestyle transformation!

CONCLUSION

Cheers to a Healthier, Happier You!

As you reach the conclusion of this juicing journey, raise a metaphorical glass to the vibrant, healthier version of yourself that you've been cultivating. The commitment you've shown to your well-being is commendable, and the positive changes you've embraced are the foundation for a more fulfilling life.

In this exploration of weight loss through juicing, you've not only discovered a plethora of delicious and nutritious recipes but also gained insights into creating sustainable habits for a healthier lifestyle. Remember, the journey doesn't end here – it's a continual process of growth and self-care.

As you move forward, carry the practical tips, diverse recipes, and personalized plans with you. Let them be the companions on your ongoing quest for well-being. Every sip of a nutrient-packed juice is a celebration of your commitment to health, and every step on this journey is a stride towards a happier you.

Whether you're sipping on a morning citrus boost, enjoying a nourishing lunch blend, or indulging in a guilt-free dessert juice, each choice is a step towards a lifestyle that supports your goals. Cherish the small victories, stay motivated through challenges, and relish the joy that comes from prioritizing your health.

Remember, this is your journey. Embrace the uniqueness of your path, and don't forget to listen to your body, mind, and heart. The journey to a healthier, happier you is an ongoing adventure, and you have the power to shape it every day.

So, here's to you – to the commitment you've made, the progress you've achieved, and the wonderful journey that lies ahead. Cheers to a healthier, happier you, and may your well-being continue to flourish in every sip and every step.